REFLECTIONS

of a

CONVOLUTED

MIND

A JOURNEY WITH MY MENTAL ILLNESS

By Dr. Samke J Ngcobo

CONTENTS

DEDICATION

Dear God, you are my sanity.

To my dear parents.

To those who have loved me beyond my struggles.

To the social outcasts who wander the streets speaking fiction, and seeing the unseen due to your mental vulnerability:
I see you. I am you and you are me.
Your silent agony has made my voice louder.

To the discipline of psychiatry and psychology: my life would be completely different without you.

To you, the reader: may your heart and mind connect with my emotional and mental vulnerability.

ACKNOWLEDGEMENTS

My Family: Unexpectedly, we embarked on a pilgrimage nineteen years ago which continues throughout our lifetime.

Ma. Baba: I would be wandering the streets aimlessly as a social outcast without you both. Your prayers have carried me through my darkest moments and your unrelenting, unconditional love and support have fostered a resilient warrior spirit within me. I stand tall with my vulnerabilities because of you both. Without you, there is no me.

Nonku. Thabile. My sisters: You mimic my bipolar illness - my best friends and worst enemies, intertwined with such intricate and intense beauty. Our relationship is complex, much like the human psyche with its glorious imperfections. Your excitement and marvel at the beauty of my dreams never ceases to humble and delight me. In this shared struggle and as a trio, we dismantled 'The Triangle'.

Ayanda Dlamini, Nare Dikgale, Lindiwe (Malindi) Khumalo-Mugabi, Yenziwe (Yenzi) Ngema, Khanya Cele, Thobile (Thobie) Nzama-Kopandru, Penny (Penns) Blose, Khin Su Le Han, Nosisa (Doro) Mbatha, Sis Lindiwe (Lindi) Xaba-Shandu, Gugulethu (Gugu) Mpanza, Zwakele Mpanza, Vuledzani (V) Munzhelele, Kusaselihle (SaMaj) Majola-Shange, Lisebo Mothepu: You remained steadfast when my mind and spirit were shattered into a million pieces. You stuck by me and lovingly pieced the fragments of my scattered sanity back together. I would be stuck in a cold isolated web of excruciating alienation had it not been for the insulated cocoon of your unconditional embrace.

Malusi Makhathini: You were warned to run away from me because I was described as mad but you bravely proceeded to gain a dear friend in me and me in you. I'm grateful that you cared enough to understand my illness and embrace me fully with it. Thank you Lusa.

Sisters For Mental Health: You died before you were born but like a phoenix, you rose from the ashes towards the colourful heavens.

Dr. Ryola Singh: Never in my life's journey did I think I would encounter a doctor of your calibre. You have remained my mental health advocate and activist when I was failing myself.

Professor Subramaney, Dr. Fiona Maynard, Dr. Friedlander, Dr. Meyer, Dr. Bokang Letlotlo, Dr. Clementine Chawane: The Doctors who respect and cherish my role as a Doctor and equally embrace the patient within me. You gave me a window to the pure and true beauty of psychiatry. My years in the psychiatry department at Wits University were rich, memorable, and meaningful because you embodied what the patient in me was seeking. Our journey continues in unison towards advocacy for mental health and for those like me.

My Dear Merle Caminsky: You continue to awaken me along the odyssey to myself.

My publisher, Grant Senzani from the Golden Goose Institute (Pty) Ltd: You guided me with such patient humility. You gave me complete and total carte blanche to independently, purposefully, and intentionally bring forth my dream to life while gently nudging me to remain on course.

Indeed, we honour the dream by doing the work.

My dear friend and cheerleader Gadifele Moeng, thank you for facilitating this classic moment of serendipity.

FOREWORD

Samke is an astronaut. A Spiritual Defier of Gravity. Where it would be the natural law for her life circumstances to bring her down and for her to stay down; she has used what she has received to hit the ground and bounce up with a force propelling her to spaces she would never have discovered. She has descended and ascended through darkness and light on our behalf and this has enabled her to have the purpose, position and passion to want to change the world one person and one perspective at a time.

I have had the privilege of being a part of Samke's mental health journey all the way from high school. It is a path that I often wanted to bump her off of because I thought it was unfair and I often asked God to just give her a break but I think it's been an adventure that, as a close friend and fellow health professional, has been important and very necessary for me. Whenever people make jeering comments about people with mental illnesses, I am able to have a reference of someone I know who has tackled Bipolar so that she has the illness and it does not have her.

I have a deep admiration and respect for my friend and I believe this book is a necessary read for everyone. It is powerful, purposeful and it will do for people what my friendship with Samke has done for me, put a face, a heart, an autonomous human with dreams and visions to mental illness. It can and it will start a rehabilitative process in our communities to understand and love those who sometimes see differently to us.

Dr. Yenziwe Ngema

INTRODUCTION

Sanity. Something so critical and delicate yet often taken for granted. Losing mental composure is like an acrobat who loses balance and falls in full view of a live audience or a musician who performs an entire concert, unaware that their microphone is switched off. It is painfully humiliating both for the individual and their loved ones.

My illness walked ahead of me. It announced itself without my consent, leaving me to deal with the unwelcome reaction of those who were unaware of its existence. Being vulnerable remains one of my life's worst fears but when I am mentally unwell,

I reside in that state and am forced to contend with its presence.

I have always been interested in understanding my mental illness and discussing issues related to mental health but my illness decided to come to the fore and prioritised itself. A myriad of questions have flooded me:

Before my birth, did I choose my illness or did my illness choose me?

Does my illness represent my bondage or my emancipation?

Would my life still be as luminous and beautiful as it is with all its scars and bruises without my mental illness? Would I like it? Would I recognise it?

The words that are enclosed in this book are for the person who is struggling mentally but is unaware of the toxicity of their thoughts as they deem it to be their baseline level of being in the world and seeing their world. I write to the individual that feels mentally confined and is unable to articulate their battle and therefore remains tormented in the abyss of confusion. I write to friends and families who are affected by the volatility of this journey and I hold hands with you in your feelings of dismay, frustration, and help-lessness.

May my offering provide you with the foresight that I have come to appreciate in hindsight. As I embark on this journey and connect with you through it, I hope that you will be refreshed by new insights about the struggles and triumphs that are in-volved in mental health related issues. May the convolutions uncoil and give you a greater sense of understanding, a deeper level of appreciation of the triumphs, and may you gain a deeper level of empathy towards the suffering which entails mental health struggles.

My offering is with the intention of creating a deeper level of understanding of mental illnesses in a vivid and relatable way. I believe that the best storyteller about mental health issues is the individual who is faced with the struggle directly. I invite you to connect and relate with my vulnerability by drawing comfort and hope from my struggles and to garner a sense of strength from my triumphs.

I have not mastered my mental illness or mental health related issues and I have not managed to master life either but what I have learned is to accept my truth and acknowledge the vulnerability that comes with being mentally ill. This has freed me and granted me peace.

Mental illnesses deserve respect and to be legitimised like every other illness. May this offering contribute to the quest of achieving this.

Chapter One
MANIA

Bipolar disorder is a type of mental illness which affects one's mood and therefore is described as a mood disorder. It typically consists of both manic and depressive episodes. Manic episodes involve elevated or irritable moods, hyperactivity, rapid speech, inflated self-esteem and a decreased need for sleep.

TOXIC HIGHS

> "Mania wasn't fun anymore.
> It wasn't creative or visionary.
> It was mean parody at best,
> a cheap chemical trick."
> **—David Lovelace—**

That insatiable thrill. The allure of possessing superpowers and feeling invincible. The seduction of no consequences. The rollercoaster that dives deep into a dark abyss and shoots up to the galaxies at bullet speed! The waterfall of tears followed by volcanic fury, raging stronger than those in a tropical island. This is how I can best describe the flood of emotions that engulf and threaten to smother me during a manic episode.

INTRODUCING MADAM J

Madam J knows no consequences. She is as fierce as a phoenix and knows no boundaries. She is dramatic and highly conceited and like a hurricane, she disrupts everything in her path. She is the friend who is unashamed to gate crash a party and subsequently hijack all the attention there. Where she passes, she is remembered. All is well when things befit her liking but when things fall apart, which they always do following her arrival, like a phantom she disappears. She is loud and unedited. She has no restraints and is blind to social cues. Her dress code is elaborate and her spending habits are equally so. Anything that is not an expensive designer label means poverty to her. Madam J has no regard or understanding of consequences.

Madam J is the name that I give to the manic episodes of my bipolar illness because Madam J is an individual and has a mind of her own. I describe her as my alter ego, my best friend, and my absolute worst enemy.

My journey with this emotional roller-coaster and mental state began nineteen years ago. This marked the start of my journey and a volatile relationship with my mental illness. My first manic episode was preceded by a depressive state. I recall being very withdrawn and would stare blankly at the television the entire day. I would refuse to engage socially and participate in sundry activities like going to the mall with my mother and sisters. All this was deemed as being part of my introversion as I was quite a shy individual. I was often described as being moody and this was not alarming as it was in keeping with my age and the expected hormonal reactions of teenagers.

Young and ill-informed as I was, I could sense something abnormal in the intensity of my emotional reactions. When upset, the intensity of my rage was insatiable and it would overwhelm me. My reactions were disproportionate to the matter at hand. My emotions led and like an ox in a ploughing field, I followed. Unbeknownst to those who stood to be affected, we were all in the eye of a great storm which would be accompanied by a downpour.

I would return from school, close the curtains and lie in bed and would think about several nonspecific things that I could not account for when I tried to recall them. My school performance was badly affected as I could not sleep through the night and therefore struggled to concentrate in class. My teachers became concerned as they noticed that the quality of my work had suddenly deteriorated. At home I withdrew further, much to the frustration of my parents. During this period, I was highly irritable, had not eaten in days, and did not sleep well. I was over-analysing things, overthinking, and I was contemplating too many things at once. People who spoke to me in person and telephonically complained that they could not follow what I was saying as I spoke too fast. Eventually, things became worse when I no longer slept at all and would pace around the house, refusing to sleep. My mental state evolved from mania and graduated to psychosis.

Mania is an exhilarating flood of emotions. The highs are incredible but the subsequent depression associated with it is equally intense and is dense. Returning from a manic episode is highly traumatic and disorienting. I always feel like I have unsteadily emerged from a deep chasm of darkness. I emerge dizzy, with no bearings to hold me in good stead. The rollercoaster comes to a screeching halt and I am flung to reality. The aftershock of the emotional earthquake makes me crave that high again. Reality is too difficult to face, whereas floating in the galaxy of carefree bliss requires no responsibility of reality which always awaits.

DEALING WITH THE AFTERMATH OF MANIC EPISODES

I have spent many years of my adult life, reeling from the reverberating consequences of previous manic episodes. The detrimental effects on my finances and subsequent psychological trauma has been difficult to process. The consequences have often led to rebounds of relapses as my appetite for any escape from reality felt like a more pleasurable remedy, although short-lived. For instance, the reckless abandon of shopping sprees and fine dining lack lustre in hindsight and are tantamount to fool's gold. At the time of these spending sprees, every item feels justified and is a desperate need.

I have spent many years of my adult life swimming upstream against a tide of financial woes in the aftermath of outrageous spending sprees garnered during my manic episodes. The rebound struggles have stressed me to a point of relapsing again as I could not cope with the strain and pressure of the financial demands. The outlandish items purchased were contradictory to anything in my reality and bank account.

I recall an experience a day after receiving my salary and already having spent all the money on outlandish, unnecessary items and landing up in a significant financial deficit before any of my monthly debit orders had been processed. To this day, seeing any form of debt gives me palpitations as I have previously landed in very distressed mental states because of the financial woes. I have had to downscale several times in order to regroup and rebuild following Madam J's dramatic arrivals and swift departures. I have nursed feelings of regret following decisions and commitments made during this state.

A manic episode does not announce its arrival; at least Madam J never does. Only those around me will note the problem but by that time, the avalanche will have collapsed.

To me, emerging from a relapse is more difficult and more exhausting than being in that state of turmoil during the actual relapse. I liken my manic episodes to a natural disaster: the episode represents a tsunami. A tsunami destroys by drowning whatever is in its path. In this case, my life is in its path. I, fortunately and as always, survive the tsunami. Life after surviving the tsunami represents my recovery phase. While I am grateful to survive the tsunami,

I do not know how or where to begin to piece the debris of my life together as so many areas of my life would have been drowned and scattered in all directions. The emotional and psychological trauma that I experience in the aftermath cannot be quantified.

The difficult thing to process about a manic episode is that, to the listener who is unaware of my mental state, everything I say sounds logical and intentional. Friends often express that they cannot gauge when I am ill as I sound coherent when I speak and am not disorganised or volatile in my behaviour. This is despite the fact that these friends, in medical practice themselves, are more used to seeing severely ill patients who are lower functioning and at the brink of being placed in placement facilities. A high functioning professional with the illness is harder to pick up on than an individual with more severe, overt symptoms.

OWNING MY IDENTITY

Madam J has been a source of great humiliation and pain. Her stubbornness and refusal to be discreet and humble has cost me greatly. Her unpredictable tendencies have left me destabilised. It's all fun and games for her when she arrives to create a circus unapologetically out of my life but the cost in the aftermath is not humorous. I have found myself reeling in agony following her arrival due to the inevitable reputational damage. I previously found myself to have been the least forgiving of her. This is because I often took blame and ownership of her behaviour, not considering that I was ill and in a relapsed state. If it was difficult for me to empathise and rationalise Madam J, how could I rationalise her with the next person and expect them to empathise?

It is difficult for people to differentiate between my true, innate beliefs and the thoughts and attention-seeking behaviours of Madam J. I would often lament and pity myself about why Madam J is an uninvited part of my life but I also realise and appreciate that I would not be the person that I am today without her. My resilience, strength, and wisdom were developed largely by her existence. My relationship with Madam J is complicated. She has presented me with many struggles but I still would not trade her for anything. Through her, I have learned to hold my head up high in the midst of the most humiliating situations. Through her, I have learned to be more resolute and to be unapologetically assertive.

My bipolar illness is a part of my identity; I cannot divorce myself from it as much as it cannot divorce itself from me. We are enmeshed in many ways but now have boundaries where it matters. I often used to describe myself as an extremist but with my journey in therapy and treatment, I have reconciled gently with myself. I am no longer a polar opposite of myself and I no longer resent Madam J due to my frustration with her behaviour. I no longer feel led by my emotions. By personifying her, my illness is given the importance and seriousness that it deserves. I did not choose her, she presented herself to me. For me to remain healthy, I have to embrace her. We are in relationship, with all the highs and lows that relationships possess. I cannot afford to see Madam J as an enemy and avoid her because this is when a volcano develops and threatens to erupt.

The Lesson: Madam J has educated me about the power which lies in owning my full, unedited story. She has taught me to embrace myself with all my flaws and to befriend those flaws instead of judging and rejecting them. She refuses to bow her head in shame of her own existence. I admire this trait as she has permitted me to allow light to shine on my vulnerabilities which in turn emancipates my mind and spirit. Hiding from our stories cripples us from living a life of substance as we are constantly trying to fix our masks which we have perfected to cover up our raw realness. Running from our stories and being ashamed of them, robs us of living with wholehearted depth and authenticity. Lacking authenticity prevents us from connecting with honest conviction both with ourselves and with others. There is no liberation in impressing others while deceiving ourselves. I am someone who values my privacy greatly, yet I have a condition that puts me in full view and under the harsh glare of scrutiny when it arrives. I have chosen to give voice and recognition to her as opposed to treating her like a deeply held secret. Secrets are cancers of the soul. Keeping my mental struggles as a secret worsens them as whenever they become exposed unintendedly, the pain and psychological damage runs deeper subsequently.

We all have struggles that we are constantly fighting and are yet to contend with, but embracing their reality and potential to teach us is what will enable us to emerge wiser and more resilient. Walking beneath, above, and around our challenges is simply delaying the inevitability of having to deal with them. Resisting or denying our painful experiences undermines our potential and abilities to overcome and rise higher in our state of being.

The rollercoaster has slowed, the thrill is calm and I live in reality. The galaxies are where they belong and I am on earth. The superpowers remain with the superheroes and I remain with my unassuming, vulnerable humanness. The volcano is a dry, aged crater and the waterfall is flowing how and where it belongs.

Madam J has been my teacher and I remain a student.

Chapter Two
PSYCHOSIS

A mental disorder that is characterised by distortions in thinking, perception, emotions, language, sense of self and behaviour. Common psychotic experiences include hallucinations (hearing, seeing or feeling things that are not there) and delusions (fixed false beliefs or suspicions that are firmly held even when there is evidence to the contrary). The ability to recognise reality and to communicate and relate with others is severely impaired. The degree of impairment is sufficient to grossly interfere with the capacity to deal with reality.

REASONING OF THE UNTAMED, CONVOLUTED MIND

"The psychotic drowns in the same waters in which the mystic swims with delight."
—Joseph Campbell—

When the mind turns on itself and threatens to destroy its very being. When it speaks in a language that only it understands, with no concern of how its words are deciphered; when it seeks to perceive an alternate reality: this is my experience of psychosis.

The inability to control my mind is a very fragile and vulnerable place to be. I am at the mercy of those around me and this unawareness is what causes stress in hindsight. A psychotic episode robs me of my dignity. It is deeply humiliating and difficult to process upon re-emergence and return to reality. Often, what I say and do in this state is judged as a truth of my beliefs and opinions. Regaining composure following a psychotic episode feels futile and is laced with feelings of defeat, shame and embarrassment.

For many, the term 'psychosis' is a confusing and poorly misunderstood term. This phenomenon is what many deem and label as madness, a deranged or unhinged mind, or simply describe as craziness. This mental state and associated behaviour often elicit fear and anxiety towards me due to the inability to rationalise my strange behaviour.

Many have read about and witnessed it but as I reflect, its complexity cannot be fully grasped unless one experiences it for themselves. If my reality in the psychotic state is of wealth, power, and prestige; the allure of this mental state seduces me to remain in this deceptive reality. When engulfed and tormented by fears of danger, my mind becomes a torture chamber with no means of escape. Both are distorted realities but one is pleasant and the other is not. I cannot tell the difference between the alternate and real.

For the observer witnessing psychosis, it is dazzling and fascinating to listen to strange words and observe odd behaviour. Some can be fascinated and find humour at witnessing this at best or are fearful and distressed at worst by the potential danger of witnessing the ill individual's detached state from reality and subsequent inability to control their behaviour. What is fiction to the listener is truth to the individual, and this conflict is what orders chaos.

MY INTRODUCTION TO THE PSYCHOTIC STATE OF BEING

Nineteen years ago, I was in the ninth grade of my schooling career. I experienced a phenomenon that was worrying to my parents, yet I was oblivious to the abnormality thereof.

I feared leaving the house because I felt watched by an invisible audience. I felt uncomfortable using my phone because I believed that my calls were being recorded. I spoke of my ability to communicate with deceased relatives and would share the messages I received from them. I deemed this to be a special gift and saw nothing wrong with this phenomenon. As the days progressed, this special gift became incredibly distressing when I started to believe that faceless and unknown people around the world could hear and listen to my thoughts. The scrutiny and ridicule of this audience was belittling. The inability to control this threatening reality was traumatic.

As I walked to the kitchen with the radio on, I believed that the people speaking through the radio were communicating with me directly. This gave me a great sense of importance and power. I soon found it highly distressing as I felt naked to the world while my thoughts laid bare for all to listen to. I felt robbed of my privacy. In the evening, I stood by the light switch. I believed that I was God and in control of the world. I believed that by simply turning on the light switch, the sun would emerge, lighting the whole world and that by switching off the light, the sun would disappear, plunging the entire world into darkness by this simple act. The light switch could control the appearance of the sun. I did not sleep the whole night as I feared that in falling asleep, I would never wake up.

The following day, my odd behaviour escalated exponentially as I was undressing and kept trying to run out of the house in that naked state. I believed that I was being held hostage in a foreign prison and needed to escape. I feared the people in the house as I believed that they wanted to harm me. My mind had become its own enemy. My bewildered and perplexed parents had reached their emotional and mental limits and decided to take me to seek professional help for the first time. This marked my first contact with mental health services. As my parents drove in pursuit of seeking medical assistance, I gazed out the window of the car, oblivious to the worry and panic surrounding me. Looking out the window, I was convinced that all the billboards depicted my life and were communicating directly with me.

Upon arrival at the waiting room of the mental health facility, I placed the magazines face down as I felt too exposed by everything depicting my life in the magazine.

Needless to say, I was admitted to the hospital. During my admission and subsequent discharge, members from my church came to see me to bring prayers and spiritual support. In the lack of understanding my mental illness for some, I was subjected to several exorcisms as I was deemed to be demon-possessed. I was avoided for fear that my demonic state was contagious. From a cultural perspective, I was believed to be bewitched and was therefore also avoided for the same reasons as by my exorcists.

This entire ordeal became an unspoken matter and was not discussed further, despite my enquiries about what had happened to me. This was so new to my parents and they themselves could not explain it to me. Following my first presentation of my illness, I remained well despite no further medical interventions. The sleeping giant remained peaceful and quiet for several years until it provoked itself and returned with its full might.

SWEET DREAM OR A BEAUTIFUL NIGHTMARE?

Being psychotic feels like a dreamy out-of-body experience. It can be a pleasant dream or it can be a nightmare. The only difference is that one does not wake up from it automatically and immediately. The extreme state of being unaware of one's surroundings can be dangerous. In extreme cases, people in this mental state have killed other people or themselves accidentally, due to confusing reality with their own perceived reality. They experience such a fear of the people around them that they try to protect themselves from the perceived threat.

During one of my previous relapses, in my psychotic state, I recall driving at high speed on an urban road with no destination in mind, out of fear that the vehicle behind me was chasing me. Here I was, crisscrossing the road before sunrise trying to escape a non-existent enemy. In hindsight and as I reflect, I recall seeing a very frightened road user who was more in fear of me than I was of them. I'm grateful that the road was quiet and that I was not harmed.

When a mentally ill person is witnessed to be speaking and behaving strangely, the lack of understanding garners a fear response by those who bear witness and understandably so. We cannot control what is unpredictable and therefore we do not know how to respond appropriately. The unfamiliar is often not welcome, especially if the unfamiliar is in the form of a person who does not understand their own behaviour due to being severely mentally unwell.

Many a time, I have wished to return to the care-free state in the aftermath of a psychotic episode. The degree of emotional and psychological burns is scorchingly painful to soothe. Being seen differently after a psychotic episode is very difficult to process. Although people may not comment about it, the screaming avoidance makes it clear that the psychotic state has become the baseline of how I'm perceived. How do people who are unfamiliar with mental illnesses rationalise bearing witness to something so extremely out of the ordinary? Life is a mystical, untamed convolution. This is what makes it the wonder and adventure that it is. Life is never static as it vibrates with dynamic aliveness. One does not need to float in a galaxy of deceptive reality because life in itself is so incredibly abstract.

The Lesson: Often as people, we wish to escape the realities of the circumstances presented to us when we are faced with adversity. We revel and feel secure in having control over ourselves, our lives, and other people. Lacking this control is terrifying. Imagine possessing no control at all but being unaware that you don't possess any of it. This is what psychosis looks like. We wish for an alternative reality when things are difficult, much like a psychotic state where things are at the mercy of what we deem to be the truth. In its very nature, psychosis is deceptive as reality is its contrast and always awaits in the shadows. Lulling ourselves into a numb comatose state is an anaesthetic against the truth. Self-deception is agreeing with a preferred truth, rejecting reality. Doing this is procrastination of the inevitable. When the mind deviates from reality, one's entire being and existence is destabilised in retaliation. Perceptions of truth are distorted and the response is equally distorted.

In some aspects, I believe that a psychotic episode is a microcosmic representation for life when it is not going our way. As much as one cannot control their behaviour during a psychotic episode, we equally cannot control the ebb and flow of life, as best as we try. Expecting that we can control it is investing in fool's gold. Embracing the unexpected is difficult but is progressive. To be perplexed and bewildered is a normal reaction but to dismiss and ignore reality breeds pathology. Being in a psychotic state has preached a symbolic sermon to my life: I should not mock or ridicule myself for a reality that I did not create, neither should I hold myself to ransom in frustration for how I react in circumstances that I did not foresee.

We spend too much time cringing with irritation towards ourselves for behaving and speaking in a manner that we cannot retract; when we cannot undo what has already been done or said. This self-deprecation is cruel and tormenting. Being gentle with our imperfections enables us to befriend them and use them as our ally. In being our ally, we are able to use the unpleasant experiences fruitfully by watering them with kindness.

I have spent many agonising moments recalling and replaying the film reel of my behaviour during my psychotic episodes. Doing this would render me despondent, defeated, and devastated. With time, I have learned to own my experience and no longer hang my head in shame or feel apologetic to those who bear witness to my behaviour. It has been a difficult journey to navigate and to make peace with. Often, I have had to wrestle with the person in the mirror and try to not be frustrated or judgemental of her. It has been difficult to reconcile that my psychotic behaviour is not me, despite the behaviour being housed in the same body. Self-judgement is worse than external judgement because like a summer's cloud, it follows you constantly. It distorts what one sees in the mirror and sparks an inappropriate reaction. I have often had to be reeled back into facing the reality of my circumstances instead of focusing on my preferences as a means of denial.

Knowing the truth of my alternate reality has freed me. Being in the realm of truth with my psychosis has exterminated the deceptive quality of the threat towards the stability of my mind. My mind is my friend and we speak the same language. Living in the realm of reality is so much safer and more stable than the unpredictable fiction presented by psychosis.

I continue to tame and rationalise the convolutions of my mind.

Chapter Three
DEPRESSION AND SUICIDE

Depression is a common mental disorder that affects mood. It is characterised by sadness, loss of interest or pleasure, loneliness, despair, feelings of guilt, or low self-worth. It also results in disturbed sleep or appetite, tiredness, and poor concentration. It results in withdrawal from social contact. At its most severe, depression can lead to suicide (the act of taking one's life).

THE DEADLY TANGO

*"Knowing your own darkness is the
best method for dealing with the
darknesses of other people."*
—Carl Jung—

The sun is my joy and depression is the eclipse. It pales everything around it with the paint of darkness. It corners one into isolation and deceives those around it.

12 years ago, I was confronted by feelings and emotions which were very new and unpleasant to me. I could not understand them, let alone articulate and rationalise them to the next person. Half-

way through studying for what is deemed to be a prestigious degree to become a medical doctor, the promise of a bright future lay ahead on the horizon. I was at the epitome of my youth, with all the dreams and expectations that were fore-casted for me just up ahead. Despite all the optimistic ideals, all I thought of and dreamt about was coffins and death. If coffins had feelings, I felt like a coffin due to the hollowness of my inner being. I had a deep-seated envy of those lying in a coffin; I craved their sleep. In my mind, those people rested in peace with no worries of the world. I was desperately in need of deep sleep due to exhaustion that I could not understand. Seeing a child cradled peace-fully is what I desperately wished for myself; my heart needed to be cradled from its despair and hopelessness. I longed for my inner being to be soothed and filled in order to drown the all-consuming emptiness.

FALLING INTO DEPRESSION

An infant's sleep was of content abandon and peaceful satiety. Infants have no care; no expectations demanded and cast upon them. I longed for this sleep so badly but could not make sense of this ominous longing. Contrary to the bright future that was forecasted for me, I could barely make it through the morning let alone face the day ahead. To think of the day ahead was a challenging enough task to consider executing. I could not think beyond moments, let alone scheduling and having to think about the weeks or months which lay before me. A feeling of dread encircled me like vultures waiting to converge towards a carcass.

I felt tightly tied to my bed by invisible ropes composed of demotivation and un-founded, insurmountable exhaustion. I found it impossible to walk and reach the knob of my bedroom door which was a mere two metres away. Bathing was too high a demand and expectation, an impossible goal to accomplish. So I resided myself to lie in bed and not bath for successive days on end, disabled by feelings of defeat and failure due to the inability to achieve simple tasks. I was disinterested in the most appealing surroundings or exciting moments and possible pleasant memories. All I wanted to do was curl up in bed with the curtains drawn in a dark room. I was oblivious to and disinterested in the most meaningful things.

I was too troubled by unrelenting guilt and shame to fall asleep yet too exhausted to stand up and face life. I could not explain or understand these feelings. My soul was as heavy as a dark block of lead. I was saturated and congested by misery yet my body felt so hollow. I was not brave enough to end it all, yet I felt like too much of a failure and coward to attempt harming myself. I perceived not ending my life as a failure. Little did I realise that it was this fear that saved me. As a result, I was followed by a dark cloud of torment in the form of suicidal thoughts. I fantasised about being hit by a bus and not survive the impact or prayed to be involved in a fatal motor vehicle accident and not make it out alive. I could hear a dark, prompting voice that was rationalising the illogical within me. From my reasoning, I would have died a more dignified death than to independently extinguish myself. That was the first time that I encountered the torment of darkness and loneliness; thoughts and feelings of craving death.

With a perceived ideal life and supportive family, how could I logically express and explain that my only wish was to simply not exist, without being judged as being ungrateful for the life that I was living. I believed that I would not be understood if I shared my struggles. Nobody would pursue the relevant help on my behalf anyway as my thoughts would not be deemed to be a disease. I did not know that I was suffering from a disease either. Mental illnesses and mental health related issues were still poorly understood or legitimised during those times. I had no idea that my thoughts and behaviour were a form of illness that could receive intervention. How could I explain my tormenting thoughts and feelings to another person when I could not understand, rationalise, or explain them to myself? Culturally and religiously, this was a sure path to hell and permanent damnation by my ancestors. This fear of grand rejection led me along a path of secrecy and silent suffering. How could I vocalise my suffering and struggle without being reprimanded and made guilty for even thinking and considering such vitriol? "How could she be so selfish?", would be the remaining begging question in my tragic absence.

UNDERSTANDING SUICIDE

Depression is a fraud and bathes in a pool of deception. Everything inside is withered, putrid weeds, deprived of sunlight yet externally it is in full bloom, emitting a fragrance so pure and alluring. It is an imposter. Nothing matters and it exists with no prospect of a tomorrow, let alone a bright one. I so desperately would crave to live the life of another; anybody's because enclosing my own soul and spirit was too overwhelming, dark, and torturous. I felt the need to empty my inner contents, haemorrhage them out and start afresh. A withered, putrid weed that could not be associated with a bright and radiant bloom felt dishonest and pretentious. It was too paradoxical and I needed to attend to it.

Suicidal thoughts and the act of attempting or committing suicide is something that is poorly understood by society at large and as a result, an individual who struggles with these thoughts and feelings is often met with disdain, scorn and judgement. We exist in a society that is obsessed with attaining eternal joy and with existing in a utopia of perfection. This expectation creates pressure which leads one to be shocked and bewildered when faced with difficulties and struggle. Any semblance of struggle is villified and frown-ed upon and it is treated as something which is alien to the human experience. This unrealistic expectation of perennial happiness is constantly pursued. To acknowledge struggle and difficulties as experiences which are a part of life is to be kinder and more compassionate towards processing difficult emotions and our human experience.

Instead of being embraced with empathy and understanding, individuals who suffer from depression and suicidal thoughts are often dismissed as selfish attention seekers who are not grateful for the gift of life. These dark thoughts are torturous. This experience is compounded by the scathing attacks which serve as a venomous poison on an already gaping wound. Succumbing to this desperate cry for help is the final scream of a tortured soul that has surrendered to defeat.

According to the World Health Organisation (WHO), it is reported that 1 person commits suicide every 40 seconds. According to global data, it occurs across the lifespan but the leading cause is between the ages of 15-29 years globally. That is one death too many. The commonly affected age group comes as no surprise to me as this is a time that is often volatile, troubled, and fragile in one's life. It is often a very noisy, crowded, yet lonely phase of life. Like dough, one is compressed and stretched by societal expectations and opinions. The other pressure comes in the form of peers. A myriad of messages threaten to pollute and engulf one's mind. For others, this life phase is a time of discovering the immense difficulties that life presents. The birth of the wounded child manifests and many do not cope and plummet into turmoil.

From a young age, we create fixed timelines for the achievement of our high goals and ambitions. These timelines exist in further rigid confines of expectations and pressure which are projected by the media and loved ones alike. As life in its unpredictable nature will have it, our plans are forced to bow down and conform to the ebb and flow of itself because life is a river that follows its own accord and dictates. We become devastated when things do not go at the pace that we envisioned and this can lead to depression and intense anxiety. Looking at those around us, we convince ourselves that they are leading better lives than we are. We tend to compare our seasons of struggle with the joyous seasons of others. This practice is bound to garner a deep sense of unworthiness and inadequacy. What we can do is plan ahead but have robust flexibility when things do not adhere to what we want at that time.

I caution us to not be so lulled into a numb slumber regarding the statistics related to depression, suicide attempts, and completed suicides. The statistics are not simply numbers; they represent people: a parent, a child, a sibling, a friend. It could be you or me. Personifying these numbers gives the statistics a greater level of depth and meaning. As a society, we tend to distance ourselves and even judge people and situations that are not on our doorstep. Until they are.

Often times, one is ashamed to vocalise the plethora of their mental struggles because of anxiety that is triggered by fear. The topic of suicide remains very taboo in the greater society and even more so in the microcosm represented by conservative communities and cultures. For as long as there is unease in confronting this issue, the precipitants will remain poorly understood and this secret suffering will persist.

The Lesson: In our current world that is filled with a plethora of distractions and escapism, it is more appealing and easier to sedate ourselves with alternative, artificial realities than to sit with pain and discomfort. Admitting to struggle and vulnerability is a very scary yet liberating thing to do. The potential risks which present themselves by being vulnerable are rejection, ridicule, and judgement. Triumph lies in relating and existing in a community that understands and shares in this struggle. The lessons which I have learned were achieved in my reflections in hindsight. My aim is to present foresight which will be a supportive tool for awareness and to legitimise this uninvited dark cloud.

Achieving eternal happiness is desired as the ultimate goal and when this does not happen, numbing ourselves with distractions becomes the easy solution. Feeling the reality of our pain and struggles is avoided at all costs. We are inundated with social media images, television shows, and advertisements that promise and lure us into believing that this is all attainable all of the time. This expectation is toxic as it leads to despondency and disappointment. We question why our lives are so ordinary and not sparkling enough when compared to the images that we are constantly flooded with.

The reality is that we will not feel inspired or inspirational all the time. Dark moments are part of our life's experience. The important thing is to differentiate between the uninspired, demotivated times of sadness, and when the darkness becomes a pathological state.

We are so much more than the books and statistics that tend to easily make us faceless and that desensitise others from our experiences. Telling our stories candidly and with conviction is an important way of providing an understanding to our loved ones and communities alike about our journey. When one is not in your shoes, it becomes difficult to understand fully what you are going through. Storytelling from our own lense is what will garner a greater level of understanding and empathy towards our journey.

A paradigm shift about depression and suicide is what will allow the rays of sunlight to overcome the eclipse, remove the dark opaque glasses, and lift one from the dark corner. It will dissolve the pallor, replace it with technicolour, and provide insulation to the lonely freeze of isolation.

Interventions will untie the tight ropes, give voice to the suffering, and provide a restful sleep that awakens one to vibrant aliveness.

Chapter Four

DOCTOR MEETS PATIENT

THE DICHOTOMY

*"Each patient carries his own doctor
inside him."*
—Norman Cousins—

I am a doctor who has patients and I am a patient who has a doctor. To amplify the reality of this dichotomy, I have been working as a mental healthcare practitioner in recent years. I am also an individual who has a mental illness; more appropriately defined, I am a mental healthcare user. This irony is something that one can perceive as a conflicting interplay of roles or glaring derision. On the contrary, these seemingly polar opposites have been incredibly beneficial and rewarding at best but devastating and disappointing at worst. I'm in a watershed space where I can observe from the perspective of a patient and the perspective of a doctor.

THE PATIENT AND THE DOCTOR

The journey of being a patient has not been an easy one. It took several years for me to eventually accept and admit to my mental illness. In my medical training, I used to see severely ill patients in the psychiatric wards and could not identify with them and their plight. They did not look like me and I therefore prejudiced against them and myself. Little did I realise that when I am ill, I behave and look like them. The scale which I used as a measuring tool was unbalanced.

Upon my first encounter with a psychiatrist nineteen years ago, I decided that I wanted to work in mental health services.

In my naïve mind, I believed that he could read my mind and I in turn wanted to develop this miraculous ability when I became an adult. With all intentions clear, my journey towards this mission began. What I did not anticipate were the hurdles, land mines, and landslides that I would encounter along this journey. I had several challenges relating to my mental wellbeing. Although my desire to become a psychiatrist was clear, I was redirected along a different path ironically because of my mental illness. As a doctor who was in a discipline in which I saw patients with mental illnesses, I have a great level of empathy and a deep sense of compassion for those like me. I have a high level of understanding of the complexities of a patient's experience with their mental illness and the myriad of factors surrounding them. I also understand the multifaceted aspects of how the illness impacts the patient and their social context and the myriad of ways in which the patient responds to the illness. We share the same health service. This connectivity has enabled me to grow in working in this field. My greatest gift is my acute awareness that contrary to the unjust stigma towards the mentally ill, I know personally what it is like to navigate this tumultuous journey.

THE UNJUST TREATMENT OF THE MENTALLY ILL

A mental illness feels, breathes, sees, tastes and has a soul. It inhabits a human being who deserves to be treated with the dignity and respect that is enjoyed by society at large. Being a mentally ill individual who is a doctor, I am well aware of my rights, availability of resources for my illness and can sense a doctor who cares.

I believe that the best storyteller about mental health related issues, is the one who is experiencing them. I also believe that the best advocate and activist for these issues is the one living with them. To share one's journey holds power. Providing a narrative for my own experiences has empowered me to stand tall and cast down the burden of shame that often comes if one's story is treated as a secret.

I learned only recently how debilitating my condition could be. Following my most recent relapse, I was placed on incapacity leave for several months in order to recuperate and return to my optimal level of functioning. Initially, I struggled with this recommendation by my doctor as I equated it to incompetency. To realise that I was not coping is something that stripped me naked of my pride and I took it very personally in a negative way. I have witnessed in my work context, patients who were being sent to placement facilities or receiving grant applications due to the disabling nature of their illness. Although I have the same condition, I did not expect such limitations to enter my life. My illness has cost me financially, emotionally, and socially. Although sharing my journey was always something that I wished to do, I did not expect for it to declare itself so loudly beyond my control. I have found this space, of sharing my story to be cathartic as I reflect and ponder about my journey thus far.

Throughout my life, I have enjoyed the luxury of private healthcare. This is a privilege that I admittedly took for granted. To be managed by a team that genuinely cares is a treasure. To be seen and valued is a right that is often treated as a favour or some form of luck. Due to unexpected financial distress which led to my most recent relapse, I found myself in a public health facility. Previously and throughout, I had always enjoyed the luxury of private healthcare, oblivious to what it is like to be in the shoes of someone receiving care in the public sector. Since qualifying as a doctor, I am fully aware of the conditions in which state facilities are, including the psychiatry departments. It is my firm belief that mental health services are highly neglected and under-resourced. Care and compassion are relative and are dependant on the individuals providing that care. During my time working in the psychiatry department, I witnessed quality patient management despite the pressures and demands that were presented and had to be dealt with. Unfortunately in the particular state hospital that I was admitted to, I became acutely aware of the attitude of staff members towards the patients that they were managing.

Apart from limited resources, I felt that the attitude was patronising, punitive and highly paternalistic. I felt robbed of my voice and freedom. I felt ignored and disregarded. I sensed that I didn't matter and was simply part of someone's job and had no personhood. I and other patients were simply seen as a collective and not as individuals who held significance and possessed some form of autonomy. The staff performed the expected, leaving their work behind. Leaving us behind. I was someone's job, not a person with thoughts, opinions and feelings. Such blatancy was palpable. In this hospital, the routine was redundant and highly unstimulating. Every day, we had to recite the date, say where we were, what the name of the hospital was, and who the heads of the ward and hospital were. The bane of my existence was shower time. Like sheep waiting to be sheered, we queued at the bathroom area where we awaited our turn to shower within thirty minutes as a collective. Furthermore, all eleven of us shared one toilet. At times, four of us would need the toilet at a time. One simply had to bear with it if the first person had needed to relieve themselves. It was worse when two people were struggling with diarrhoea at the same time; which was the case during my admission. A simple request for toilet paper was met with irritation by the nursing staff and security who had divided the toilet paper into pieces. The remainder of the day was left for us to graze in the dining hall area or to sleep out of sheer boredom at 11 am.

The occupational therapy service that was offered was too basic to participate in in terms of the activities that were offered. As a result, I attended once and did not return. I had also declined to be seen by the therapist offered as I clearly informed the team that I had my own therapist of three years. I soon realised that I had become a nuisance in the ward. My defiance, assertiveness and retaliations at several ludicrous and unfounded rules were becoming increasingly irritating to the team and I was met with equally increasing hostility. Having my own voice was rejected as I had to conform to the thinking and reasoning of others. The treating psychiatrist at the facility was made aware of what they deemed to be disruptive behaviour, so I soon became a nuisance to her as well. Her attitude of disdain towards me was palpable. I tried my utmost to express my frustrations and it clearly fell on deaf ears and deliberately so. I found her to be harsh, uncaring and dismissive. It was obvious that she found me to be arrogant and perceived me as the misbehaved patient who was demanding special treatment. It did not help that the ward knew about my profession as a doctor. The staff felt challenged and did not like it. For this, they had to put me in my place.

She had my career capabilities put into question, despite only managing me for two weeks and having no documented background regarding my work performance at all. No formal assessments were performed by the managing team in the ward to determine my suitability to continue in my position as a fully functional doctor. Her opinion and judgement of me were both based on my ill state which was not my baseline level of functioning. It was, therefore, a biased and prejudiced assessment. I have never been met by such hostility and irritation from a healthcare provider. I recall her expressing that I was wasting time during one of her ward rounds as she had other patients to see. I was refusing to leave the room and she instructed the nurse to call the next patient in while I was still in the consultation room and still speaking to her. Her tone and expressions towards me were so obvious of dislike. Whenever I enquired about the justification for the prolonged admission, I kept getting responses related to standard procedure.

My defiance and assertiveness were perceived as arrogance. I recall being warned by nursing staff to behave myself if I wanted to be discharged. On the third and last week of my admission, I obeyed this absurd instruction by remaining quiet and largely incognito and as sure as clockwork, my 'good behaviour' granted me a discharge. There were so many breaches of confidentiality and privacy as many of the doctors who were managing me were people that previously attended university with me. I soon became a topic of discussion amongst them, to a point that people from outside contacted me and informed me about their knowledge of who my treating doctor was, following my discharge. It seems that when one is mentally unwell, their intellect is often simultaneously put into question and undermined.

Following my discharge, I left that hospital more mentally and emotionally traumatised than upon my arrival. In life, we all want to be seen, heard, and to feel like we matter. I was well aware during this admission that none of that existed. I had to relinquish my rights and freedom which I constantly tried to preserve through my vocal protests and defiance. I still cannot understand why I was admitted for as long as I was, only to receive medication with no ward programme at all to occupy and stimulate me. The nothingness of every day and lack of stimulation was dulling to the mind and rendered me sluggish. It undermined my capabilities and intelligence. Just because I was unwell mentally, it did not mean that I was not aware of my surroundings and the inappropriate way in which things were being done and in how I was being treated.

The Lesson: The terrible experience of the unwarranted, unjust treatment in that hospital and the resultant fury, birthed an activist and advocate in me to stand in the frontline on behalf of those like me who have mental illnesses but have no voice or are unaware of the power which lies in their voices. I believe that there is no better advocacy than self-advocacy. Many can support the cause of the mentally ill but only we can shout loudest and be heard as our mental scars make us invisible to those who choose not to see or listen. It is critical to not rob us of any semblance of autonomy and a sense of personhood. Autonomy is not a priviledge to negotiate or a reward for good behaviour; it is a right. It is this lack of empathy and compassion that serves as the root cause of stigma and perpetuates the ignorance of those who do not understand mental health related issues and the journey of the mentally ill.

My illness has been my teacher in my journey as a doctor. It has enabled me to have a background understanding of the life of those who share about their journey with their mental illness. I am a better doctor because of my struggles. Some things are not taught in the lecture hall but are taught by life itself. Most of the skills that I have attained to navigate life were not obtained from those teaching me but by my struggles themselves which have taught me humility and empathy towards the life of others. As a doctor, my illness informs me not to look at a patient solely as the bearer of disease but as someone who engages and operates in an ecosystem of being as an employee, a parent, a sibling, a friend, and a contributing member of society.

I have a doctor who genuinely cares and sees me as a person with legitimate thoughts and feelings. My experiences were validated and I have a voice and authority in how I am managed with my illness. Through my doctor, I met someone who I was inspired to become when managing my own patients. The way she cares for me is in such contrast to what I experienced during my admission to that particular hospital. I became aware of the autocratic manner in the way in which I was treated there because I knew and was familiar with my rights and was familiar with the respect with which I was used to being treated. Being mentally unwell does not equate brainlessness, yet the attitude towards the mentally ill screams and re-enforces that perception. Mental wellbeing is not for the chosen few, it is a human right.

In being a doctor, I met myself. In meeting myself, I met my doctor.

Chapter Five
STIGMA

Negative feelings that people have about particular circumstances or characteristics that someone may have.

PUNISHMENT
FOR AN UNCOMMITTED SIN

*"What we don't need in the midst of
struggle is shame for being human."*
—Brene Brown—

Imagine a young man who collapses to the ground and is convulsing. He foams at the mouth and defaecates on himself. Imagine someone standing over this person, jeering and laughing at him. Imagine observing an elderly woman who falls off her wheelchair and lies helplessly contorted on the floor. Imagine children hovering over her, imitating and mocking her state of vulnerability on the floor. None of those situations would elicit humour and those who ridicule and find humour would be met by disdain and disapproval.

In a state of confusion, a man strips naked in public and points and argues with the sky. This man is met by fear, judgement, and ridicule. Like this man, in a disinhibited state of illness, I screamed publicly on a social media platform, made scathing remarks, and spewed threatening nonsensical proclamations. The audios circulated throughout my work setting and I became a source of gossip, secret labelling, and humour. This is what stigma looks like.

We all know the feeling of being vulnerable, yet oftentimes there is very little empathy and compassion towards each other when in this state. The seat of judgement and detachment feels more comfortable. There is a special kind of icy and raw pain that is experienced when being ridiculed and feeling humiliated. The searing, inconsolable pain of the spirit from a heart that has been seared by damnation and judgement can be unbearable. The agony of alienation and isolation from being misunderstood, feeling exposed, and enveloped by shame is excruciating. I could never fully relate or empathise with the sting and throbbing pain of experiencing stigma until I found myself bare in my vulnerability under the harsh glare of the microscope of human judgement and opinion.

AND ALONG CAME DISGRACE

What makes stigma more remote and different from the exposure of a grave mistake made in public, is that one has no intention attached to it and it is uncontrollable, while the other is avoidable. My experience of being stigmatised was different from feeling offended by other people's reactions because instead of feeling offended, one is perceived as an offensive, pungent, intrusive odour.

I developed my mental illness long before mental health- related issues had gained the recognition that they do at this present time. I recall in earlier years when I would relapse and church members would come to pray for me during this period. Although the prayers were welcomed and helpful, the cost was that they were accompanied by fear as many could not understand my mental illness and dismissed me as demon-possessed. Their growing discomfort meant that when they came to pray, they refused to consume anything that was offered by us in the form of food and beverages. In ignorance, they feared that my behaviour would be contagious and could be transmitted to them. A lack of understanding was to blame as they were unfamiliar with what they were witnessing and were bewildered as a result. I, on the other hand, had to deal with the rejection and judgement for this uncommitted sin.

Being a victim of stigma is a lonely place. In experiencing it, one loses trust for people and subsequently becomes withdrawn. Although I have relapsed several times previously, my most recent relapse occurred on a public platform, leaving me like a shrivelled prune of excruciating shame, pain, and humiliation. The feeling of being bare was much like a pruned green twig exposed to the unrelenting heat of the African sun. The pain was crippling and it glared. The pain of humiliation would wake me up and threaten to drown me in a pool of tears. It would sedate me with utter emotional exhaustion. My entire body ached. People distanced themselves from me as they did not know how to react to me. I was seen through the lens of my ill state; which is one of vulnerability. Due to feelings of being self-conscious, I withdrew and distanced myself in order to regroup in a private, safe and embracing space.

I liken my most recent relapse as the inevitable sinking of the Titanic and I found that people rummaged furiously to jump off the ship. I represented the ship. Jumping off in avoidance seemed to be the more logical and safer option than to sink along with me because my mental plummet was inevitable. Jumping off and swimming to shore had the promise of a better outcome. Associating with me was a contagious disease and a surge of rejection permeated. I felt isolated.

The humiliation and trauma that I experience in the aftermath of a relapse is always psychologically damaging and emotionally crippling. It feels as if I need to redeem myself for an uncommitted sin. There are feelings of defeat involved, coupled with the hypersensitivity towards people's perceptions and opinions of me. It is an incredibly difficult journey to navigate. As a medical professional who has worked for mental health services, I have been privy to the candid, unedited thoughts of senior and junior doctors, and contemporaries alike. I have been privy to the comments made about mentally ill patients by the same people who treat them. A colleague once expressed how funny she found 'these people'. Unbeknownst to her, I was and remain one of 'those people'.

I recall being approached in the parking lot by one of the senior doctors who informed me, unprovoked, that she knew that I have a mental illness and went on to inform me which of her colleagues had told her of my diagnosis. She spoke as if she was privy to a dark secret that I was hiding. This same doctor often took liberties to disclose the diagnoses of other doctors to junior colleagues as well. An aura of discomfort diffused as confidentiality was blatantly being breached by someone who should have known better and whom I expected to be exemplary.

Media outlets have often not been helpful in their portrayal of the mentally ill and the role of mental healthcare providers. As a result, discrimination is perpetuated by this ignorance and lack of sensitivity.

ERADICATING THE SCOURGE OF STIGMA: FROM WITHOUT AND WITHIN

In recent years, the advent of the mental health movement, as I describe it, has been progressive with regards to legitimising mental illnesses and shining the spotlight on mental health related issues. Despite this, there is still a paucity of knowledge and understanding of the experience of individuals who struggle with mental health issues. I deliberately choose to shy away from describing myself as someone who suffers from a mental illness. I own my journey and am not a victim of it. Seeing myself as a victim or sufferer is a way of conceding defeat and stigmatising myself. My illness comes with many challenges which I acknowledge and have come to accept.

As a society, we have come a long way in understanding mental illnesses and matters surrounding mental health, although we need to run in faster strides as there is still a long way to go. Normalising mental health issues is the first step in eradicating the scourge of stigma. Like a birth defect or physical disability that is acquired during one's life journey, a mentally ill person does not choose this invisible struggle. Speaking publicly about my mental health issues is my attempt to dispel stereotypes about those like me and to educate those who do not understand this journey. I'm often told that I do not look like someone who has a mental illness. This is why I choose to openly embrace my reality in order to dispel this stereotyping of what is expected from a mentally ill individual. I owned my reality early on in order to control my own narrative. Despite this, I still experienced what was previously an abstract concept.

Exposure to stigma and the subsequent feeling of loneliness due to being rejected makes the experience of shame and alienation worse. As humans, we are all flawed. By simply existing on this earth, we will inevitably stumble or cause others to stumble either wittingly or unwittingly. What inspires us to rise again, is the warm embrace of grace, compassion and empathy. I have learned that the greatest and most powerful form of empathy is the one that is afforded to oneself. I cannot control or manipulate how people perceive me during or after my state of vulnerability but I can control how I perceive myself. Doing this with sincere conviction and genuineness is sheer liberation. In the aftermath of a relapse, I often find myself cringingly shrunk and curled into a tight entanglement because I was concerned about what others thought of me. This in itself is a self-inflicted and self-defeating prison with inevitable adversity and un-necessary suffering.

As I continue to address and challenge the stigma of the public about mental illnesses and the mentally ill, I simultane-ously continue to wrestle fiercely with my own stigma towards myself. I deal with it by forgiving and embracing my humanness. I believe that having mercy towards one's self enables one to embrace the human-ness of another. The lack of tolerance for others is a sign of lack of tolerance to oneself and it is an unnecessarily heavy burden to carry. To embrace, forgive and have grace towards the struggles of others, is to embrace, forgive, and have grace for oneself. I find it difficult at times to provide that kindness to myself. This reality is paradoxical as while I fight others against stigma, at times my own mind becomes an enemy unto itself due to the nature of my illness. The reality is that while we wish to live inspired and to inspire others, it is not a perennial reality. Days of discouragement are a reality. A mental issue compounds those life challenges.

We do not choose the set of circumstances which belie and intercept us, neither can we control the reaction of those who bear witness to those circumstances. What we do have control over, is how we respond and make use of that situation positively. We live in a society that embraces conformity and one which rejects otherness. The unique and extraordinary elicits discomfort and is therefore shunned. The predictable and familiar feels safer and is, therefore, easier to manage and control. At a large scale, this is what leads to wars and at a microcosmic level, to victimisation and harming of others socially.

Stigma is a reflection of one's discomfort with aspects of themself because it expresses itself when something within feels threatened. The unfamiliar elicits anxiety as something is triggered, something fearful from within. This is why there is a strong need to educate people in order to counter this reaction.

The excruciating pain of stigma has served as the bedrock from which I was catapulted to rise. I have developed an unrelenting level of resilience that I have a great appreciation for. It was painful to recall the public display of my illness. It came unannounced and arrogantly paraded to make itself known. I believe that sharing my struggle will serve as a catharsis and comfort to the individual who finds themself in this position as they can relate and have hope. Seeing through the lens of prejudice is limiting as the person being looked at is not seen wholistically but instead is seen through a bias. I have had to grapple with reputational damage as my relapse clouded an objective view of who I am and what I stand for.

The Lesson: We live in a society that shuns any form of struggle and worships those who are already triumphant, neglecting the odds they had to face. The chapter of struggle is often overlooked in the haste to celebrate the phase of overcoming. I challenge us to embrace the time of struggle as this is what shapes us to become better people. Resilience is not fostered during easy times. Sitting with difficult emotions is something that we prefer to escape because of the agony that they present. What we fail to realise is that on the other side of these emotions is where victory awaits. The only way beyond our pain is to go through it.

In the aftermath of my relapse, I so desperately wanted to sleep it away and wake up from the nightmare. Unfortunately, I could not wake up from reality no matter how much I desperately tried to wish it away. Day in and day out, I kept waking up and was stalked by recollections of the incident. My body ached; I could not divorce myself from the humiliation. I felt abandoned and forgotten. I felt that any credibility I had prior to my relapse was obliterated. Any form of composure or restraint that I was known for, fell away and my identity became the illness. I was disappointed to learn that some of my colleagues who work within the discipline related to mental health found humour in my experience. The greatest disappointment was that I expected a greater level of empathy and understanding from people who see patients who share in my struggle. In hindsight, I'm grateful to have become an example who has decided to vocally stand up and shine a light on the experience of being on the other end of the spectrum as a patient

I now sit in my lab, glaring through the lens of my microscope and analysing the reality of those who still subject the mentally ill to stigma and the mediums which still perpetuate the narrative of discrimination. The African sun has strengthened the twig which is now browned and solidified by the pain which in turn has fostered resilience and wisdom. I am no longer lame and crippled by shame from my relapse; I am standing tall with strength and authority. Like a gentle balm, my heart is consoled and no longer aching from humiliation as I am celebrating the strength which lies in my vulnerability. I am no longer seared or alienated for I am cele-brating my voice in the midst of those who share in the same struggle.

The shame, trauma and self-doubt have been exorcised. I have been atoned from my uncommitted sin.

Chapter Six

TREATMENT

A HARD PILL TO SWALLOW

"The person who takes medicine
must recover twice: once from the
disease and once from the medicine."
—Dr. William Osler—

The journey of taking treatment is an arduous road to navigate. The issues impacting how one takes treatment and the struggles thereof, are a multifaceted mosaic that outnumbers those found in a Roman Cathedral. The realm of treatment should not be merely simplified to the swallowing of pills. A patient exists in an ecosystem that has to function synergistically like a well-oiled machine. My spiritual foundation, my loved ones, my psychiatrist, my psychologist and occupational therapist have been critical in my journey of sustained mental wellbeing. Non-adherence to treatment should not be simplified and reduced to a deliberate act of self- sabotage or negligence. A myriad of factors have influenced my commitment to taking treatment. It is important to understand those influences in order to help in supporting someone who struggles with these issues.

THE ECOSYSTEM

In the ecosystem which facilitates my mental wellbeing, I am central in an electric network that consists of my loved ones, my spiritual life and the intervention of my multidisciplinary team. These electric feeds are symbiotic and exist for my benefit.

SPIRITUALITY

It has taken me many years, and kinder experiences, to learn that my spiritual life is not in conflict with my mental stability. These two entities were in intense conflict earlier on in my illness when I was growing up. To be described as demon-possessed and therefore blamed for my illness was highly psychologically damaging. Which doorway had I created or what act had I performed that attracted demons to find a nurturing home in me? These questions and feelings of rejection tormented me. Why did God create a home in me to house demons? What in me needed to be exorcised? How was I the weakest link in my family? What supplications did I fail to say and what deeds did I fail to do? How could I remedy my lack of faith and belief? My fourteen-year-old mind was riddled with confusion and guilt. I was the agent of evil and chaos that had befallen the life of my family. Why me?

Nobody understood what was happening to me, so nobody was able to calm my anxiety or soothe my distress. If God housed demons in me, I in turn, did not want any room in His house. My exorcists were afraid to drink and share meals and beverages which we offered from my home. It became a point of discussion that there were evil spirits in my home which entered through me. My existence was a conduit for evil as evidenced by my strange behaviour. With time and growth, I learnt that these attitudes and belief systems were fueled by a lack of understanding.

My spirituality is not a substitute for taking treatment, and equally my treatment is not a substitute for my spirituality. I was born with a chemical imbalance that influences my mood and behaviours. To create spiritual calm and balance, I take medication religiously. My spirituality has enabled me to rationalise and make peace with my mental illness. A sense of peace and calm is the compass from within, which informs me of my mental state. A lack of calm and peace is the alarm bell that signals trouble. My illness has presented itself as a blessing in disguise and even though it comes with several challenges, I would not pray it away. My illness has led me to myself. I would not possess the depth of knowledge and empathy towards the struggles and vulner-abilities of others had my life not collapsed as many times as it has. Finding strength in my vulnerabilities was birthed through rising from them. My life is laced with greater meaning because of my difficult experiences. My pain has birthed a greater level of compassion of others and I know full well that I would not possess enough of it if I did not have my mental illness.

LOVED ONES

My family and those close to my family have been critical in my journey towards my consistent mental wellbeing. The support and understanding of loved ones have no substitute. To be loved and embraced after a relapse is a balm to a rotten wound. To still be seen as myself and lacking nothing is therapeutic. The suffering and impact of my illness on my loved ones is something that I have often underestimated. With deeper reflection, I have managed to stand in their shoes and watch helplessly with them as they see and hear me out of control; unable to stop me from talking, unable to normalise my outrageous behaviour. To visit me in hospital and see other ill patients who were equally highly disinhibited; to await security to call me from my room. Nobody wants to visit their loved one in hospital, especially in a mental institution which remains engulfed by stigma. Their worry about my safety whilst in the psychiatric ward with people who were equally unable to control their own thoughts and behaviours must have been difficult. The experience is equally traumatising for loved ones who oftentimes are more affected whilst I am drunk with psychosis. They experience reality with no pause while I float in my dreamy state.

Through them, I have become aware of how much my wellbeing means to them. My mental illness does not belong to me alone, it is a disease carried by those who are connected to me. I have become more sensitive and have realised that my relapses are not solely about me and therefore, the pain is not felt solely by me. My mental health issues affect the psyche of those in and around me and this influences my need for continued sanity.

MULTIDISCIPLINARY TEAM

My psychiatrist and psychologist have been critical in my mental health journey. In a world which still cannot differentiate between the two roles, I have found much-needed nurturance in both of them. We live in a society that frowns at needing and seeking help. Showing any form of need is a sign of vulnerability which is dismissed as weakness; for which there is no room. One buckles under the pressure of having to keep all aspects of life in pristine order and simultaneously so. I was one of those people who sought pride in wanting to be needed and denied any need for support. Being aware of my mental illness, it became paramount to keep all areas of my life pristine, hence I would overcompensate in my various life roles. I wanted to be the best to everyone and everything, except to myself. This left me depleted and resentful. This self-defeating exercise would constantly lead to me relapsing.

My saving grace has been my psychiatrist and psychologist who respected my autonomy and rationalised my problem in my thoughts which influenced my moods and behaviour patterns. It took several rock-bottom moments to reach my final turning point. The cost of the relapse was too high. Picking up the pieces in the aftermath was an avoidable disruption. The feelings of defeat were enough proof that I needed help. I liken the journey of taking treatment to the grieving process. I have grieved and have come to terms with the fact that my life will not flow independently without it. This has been a large, hard, and bitter pill to swallow.

DENIAL

Coming to terms with my illness was not an overnight reality. Denial has been one of the greatest demons that I have had to contend against because I was unaware of any abnormalities in my reactions or behaviours.

My relationship with my medication is a complex one. It was initially very tumultuous but it has improved with time. I would tower over the medication with resentment and snarl at it with sheer resentment. I used to ask myself why I needed treatment to keep well when others did not. Why did I have a chemical imbalance needing medication to keep my moods in equilibrium and keep my mind stable? At times I questioned how and why I possessed a chemical imbalance innately and therefore required external means to correct it. It simply did not make sense to me. It scared me to be informed that my sanity lay in the hands of means that I did not arrive to earth with but had to depend upon. The medication seemed to know my dependency on it as it always waited patiently for my return no matter how often I dismissed its importance or rejected it. In total denial of my condition, I would blatantly reject it and absolve myself from the reality and responsibility of needing it. As a result, I would relapse due to refusing to accept my need to take the treatment. Like a tormented lover in a toxic relationship, I would begrudgingly return to my medication that knowingly and patiently awaited my return. I have attempted one too many times to shy away from this firm and sobering reality of needing to take my medication.

It has been exhausting to frequently have to collect the debris of my life following a relapse.

ANGER

I have wrestled with feelings of anger and resentment towards my illness and those who believed that I have the illness. I simply could not understand what was peculiar in my behaviour that would render me mentally unwell and warrant treatment. What was so out of the ordinary in my words and actions? What made me different from others when not on the prescribed treatment? I was overcome by furious frustration. It angered me that I needed medication to remedy what was deemed to be peculiar. I saw nothing peculiar in my moods and behaviours, therefore I felt deeply offended.

Adverse reactions to treatment have often been discouraging in my journey of taking medication. Although the treatment balances my mind, in retaliation to this, my brain dulls itself in an act of defiance. Consequently, this stand-off tends to impair my ability to concentrate, retain information and recall it. In frustration, I would join this protest of my mind by defaulting treatment.

It angered me that I needed treatment which in turn also made me ill. I struggled with the shaking of my hands and had difficulty writing as a result. My tertiary years of study were difficult as I was riddled with struggles relating to medication. Significant weight gain has been a disfiguring conundrum. I gained weight exponentially within a space of four months. This was devastating as it negatively affected my self-esteem. As the dosing of my medication was on the increase, my work performance was deteriorating when being required to work overnight being on call.

In addition to this, the cost factor needs to be taken into consideration. The treatment is expensive and some of it is not covered by the medical aid. What helped me accept and make peace with taking treatment was realising the consistent negative aftermath of not taking it. The consequences of not taking treatment were and remain too high a price to pay.

BARGAINING

I have often tried to find alternative ways of addressing my issues related to my illness. I simply could not fathom that I had a problem and as a result, I would secretly gamble my health to see for how long and how far I could function without the treatment. I used to overcompensate by biting off more than I could chew, with the aims of concealing the fact that I had mental limitations. I subjected myself to my own stigma. The treatment was always warranted, yet I somehow convinced myself otherwise. I was convinced that my mental illness was a fallacy, much to the frustration of my loved ones.

DEPRESSION

I used to personalise having a mental illness and blamed myself for having it. I struggled to separate myself from the fact that I did not ask to have it nor did I orchestrate the aftermath of a relapse. Like porous soil, I absorbed the flood of stigma and judgement, leaving me emotionally feeble.

ACCEPTANCE

It is difficult when the saviour is an enemy simultaneously. How can I hate something that only comes with good intentions? Having a need and admitting to it is a difficult place to be. It is a vulnerable and fragile place to find oneself. Coming to terms with the truth of my reality has been difficult to make peace with but has definitely been worth it. Realising that taking treatment is my own responsibility for my well being has been sobering.

Within these complex issues, a feeling of gratitude is perennial as I am aware that without the treatment and multidisciplinary management, my life would be completely different and poorly functioning without the available treatment modalities. The grief has brought me my healing in the form of a sound mind. My act of surrender is what brought my emancipation.

My mental ecosystem flows synergistically with vibrant delight.

EPILOGUE

*"There is a secret strength that
vulnerability knows."*
—Timothy Shriver—

My nineteen-year pilgrimage has brought me to this point. It has been nothing short of an adventure with no glamour but one that has been a colourful, glorious and beautifully packaged mess. My mind has betrayed me many times but has been my ally for most of it.

To my fellow champions who fight what is meant to dismantle us, let us continue to own the fragments of our sanity and sing a song of hope in unison. To those who love us through this struggle and soldier on with us, it is my hope that my reflections have garnered a greater sense of hope and encouragement. We will conquer as we charter this often murky territory.

What a mysterious wonder it is to be human. The convoluted mind stands watching its reflection and sees simple sanity.

ABOUT THE AUTHOR

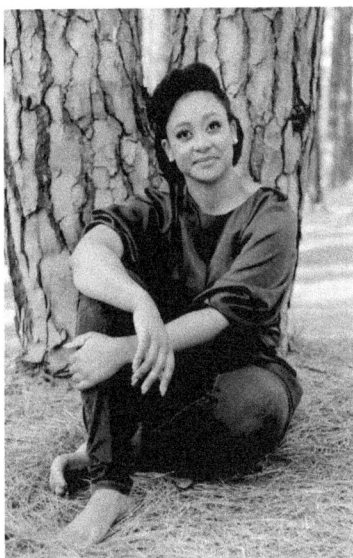

Dr. Samke J. Ngcobo is a medical doctor who was born and raised in Durban, KwaZulu-Natal. She is currently based in Johannesburg.

She has lived with Bipolar Disorder, a mental illness which she was diagnosed with at the age of fourteen. Her illness came at a time when mental illnesses were poorly understood and therefore not embraced, leading to stigma and judgement. After several unpleasant experiences related to her mental illness, she realised the importance of advocacy and activism on behalf of the mentally ill.

Dr. Ngcobo is an author, philanthropist, professional speaker, and entrepreneur. She founded a non-profit organisation called Sisters For Mental Health which aims to collaborate with other organisations that relate to mental health and mental illnesses. She also founded a company called Vocal Mentality (Pty) Ltd which focuses on psycho-educating the corporate community and community at large about mental illnesses and mental health.

Her dream is to wake up to a day when mental illnesses are seen for the legitimate illnesses that they are. She continues to champion the fight against stigma through vivid storytelling and teaching society about the journey of those who struggle with mental illnesses.

Check out our website for more information:

www.sistersformentalhealth.co.za
www.vocalmentality.com

Connect with us on social media:

1. Instagram: @_vocalmentality
2. Instagram: @sistersformentalhealth

www.ingramcontent.com/pod-product-compliance
Lightning Source LLC
Chambersburg PA
CBHW032007190326
41520CB00007B/388